Got Sugar?

Philosophy of a Sweet Tooth

Comprehensive Lifestyle Guide
For All of Life's Delicious Journeys

Debbie Markham

Note

The information in this book is believed to be accurate and true at the time of printing. The author can not accept any legal responsibility of liability for any errors or omissions that may be made nor for any inaccuracies nor for any harm or injury that comes about from following ideas in this book.

Comments welcomed:
debbie@functionablyhappy.com

To Nate and Zoe who inspire me everyday.

And to everyone who has positively influenced me in my constant quest to turn obstacles into enriching experiences, thank you.

Embarking on this journey of life is way more fun sharing ideas, facing challenges and brainstorming amusing solutions with all of you!

Table of Contents

Chapter Two:

Lifestyle Tips and Tricks

FORWARD

Many who have eaten my brownies, cereal treats, and other sweet delights have gone on to lead normal lives, enjoyably!

All joking aside, this book is not intended as medical advice. I'm neither a doctor nor a dietitian. For 25 years I've been soaking up health and fitness information like a sponge cake! There is so much written on diet, health, and exercise, and let me tell you, I've read it all.

It all began with a few file folders: one for recipes, another for diet and health, and the last for fitness and exercise plans. Before I knew it, I had accumulated a lot of sweet material. Through all this I learned that it is possible to maintain a healthy, strong physique while enjoying sweets daily! So, here, I want to share my lifestyle tips on doing it all, enjoying it all, having my cake, and eating it too.

The following is a collection of the best ideas from those file folders sprinkled with my own sweet philosophy on exercise, diet, stress, fun and life.

Bon Appetit!

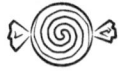

Introduction

"Sugar is the sun's energy stored in a tasty package."

My active lifestyle requires knowledge of what's best for my body. That said, I really enjoy life more with sugar. So I've decided to ride the line between healthy and unhealthy. Allowing myself to eat sugary things reminds me of my youth which makes me happy. I like to add elements of health to the desserts and baked goods I create; this way I still feel like a kid and can feel somewhat responsible too. For you, I want to be the voice of sugar-reason.

Many days I eat on the run—an apple fritter for breakfast, a granola bar for lunch, some pizza and beer for dinner. But that same week I'll do a 180—a fried mix of one egg and three egg whites breakfast, a salad for lunch, a dish of grilled fish and veggies for dinner.

Embracing my busy life, and accepting that I'll eat less nutritiously at times, knowing I'll flip back to my healthy ways, has made me mentally comfortable. In the back of my mind I'm always carving out time to be in the kitchen mixing, loving, and sharing delicious recipes.

Most diets fail because they neglect to address healthy ways of consuming sugar. I'm all about a lifestyle that supports balance. But remember, balance is a journey.

So there you have it, it's not an option for me to give up sugar. It's a matter of increasing components of health and exercise to balance out sugar consumption. It's about relaxing a bit, enjoying a perfect cake for all the individual components that are needed to create it. Thinking like this reminds me of all the sweet, rich, healthy, salty, dry, solid members of my family, and how each one, although unique, is needed to create our beautiful family tree.

I started compiling all this information in a book for myself once three messy file folders reached maximum capacity. Referencing them each week had become a nuisance rather than something I looked forward to when searching for ideas. Because it was rewarding to work towards accomplishing this task, completing this book, I dove in and never looked back.

As I told friends, they too were excited to see what I did to stay strong. It's hard to say if those closest to me were supporting me out of obligation or true interest, but either way, I thought, I'm going to write this for all the sweet tooths out there who are tired of reading the perfectly balanced daily menus that lack sugar!

As scared as I was to present my ideas, my genuine interest to just write what I know guided me. Over the years I've made lots of small, fun changes in my personal lifestyle. And I continue to look for silly ways to make me smile throughout my chore-filled, responsibility-packed days. Over time, I honed in on what things were doable on a regular basis, things that motivated me daily and helped me truly enjoy waking up each morning!

This book shares my habits (both healthy and indulgent), my mentality, and my observations which have really helped me squeeze all that great nectar out of life. I'm just an average girl who loves to eat good-tasting food as well as feel strong and healthy.

I encompass a love of all sports. I'm a curious reader of health and fitness trends. I frequent group exercise classes like yoga, Pilates, and pump it. I also practice solo-training (including training for triathlons and running races) and have qualified for the Boston Marathon. With insight from doctors and chiropractors, as well as physical and family therapists, I've gathered some great tips on keeping active and healthy. I'm also competitive—to the point where I find that making a game out of every workout, chore, or meal makes it more interesting! The underlying intent of my lifestyle is to have fun. And I do it while staying healthy and strong, and indulging my sweet tooth's desires.

While many nutritionists and trainers agree with various aspects of my healthy and sugar-filled lifestyle, some may not subscribe entirely to my interpretation of living the sweet life.

Experience it for yourself—see if you too squeeze all the sweetness of life, in every way possible!

Chapter One:

Cultivate a Healthy Mind

Acquire Knowledge

I enjoy the challenge of maintaining my weight in a world of increasingly delicious food and desserts. Knowledge fuels confidence, so I investigate vitamins, ingredients, calories and nutritional content of foods and watch what I eat. I also talk to people who know more than me and read anything (articles, brochures and books) relating to a lifestyle of health, strength, organization, and happiness.

There are many components to knowledge. Knowing oneself, knowing actual information, and also knowing how and when to use or share the information to inspire positive changes!

We all monitor our money daily, we constantly think of how we're going to spend it. We also plan how and when to save it, how to use it and where to donate it. It's the same with staying fit. Keeping track of what I eat reminds me of my bank account. I don't think of it as a chore or an annoyance, I think of it as being smart so I can enjoy indulgences without stress. This is a game I know works for me.

For example, by reading Starbucks' Nutrition by the Plate pamphlet as I wait in line, I know how to balance out my choices for the rest of the day, or how to order in the future when in a hurry. I was surprised and very excited to learn an apple fritter doughnut is similar in calories and fat to a zucchini muffin! This knowledge allows me to enjoy eating apple fritters, and helps me plan to eat veggies and protein for dinner!

Another example is realizing that one cup of Raisin Bran has approximately the same amount of calories and sugar as a Pop Tart or Take 5 candy bar. Cereal and Pop Tarts are fortified with vitamins, all three have the same protein and the cereal has the most fiber. But if I've eaten some whole grain bread and veggies for fiber, and taken my vitamin, I feel okay eating a Take 5 Bar or Pop Tart for dessert.

You can to gain more knowledge like this by reading online. Try to learn by reading online. A handy web site is http://nutrition.about.com/od/changeyourdiet/a/

calguide.htm. Type in height, weight, age and it shows your caloric needs. Another great way to learn is by using iPhone Apps. *Calorie Counter and Diet Tracker by MyFitnessPal* can help you stay aware of calories.

Research shows that people overestimate how many calories they burn during exercise. So, in order to avoid this miscalculation, I've learned how many calories different activities use and keep it in mind. I found some charts online stating the calories burned per exercise and duration. To find similar calorie-burning charts, type in 'exercise calorie calculator' into your favorite search engine. These charts are great because they take into consideration your weight. When I plugged in 200 lbs for 30 minutes of jogging, the internet chart said I burned 300 calories. When I input 130 lbs for 30 minutes of jogging, it said 200 calories were burned. Since treadmills don't consider weight, the calories they suggest being burned don't seem accurate.

I'm proud of my healthy eating habits. I feel I've accomplished something and then I'm excited to indulge in a treat because I earned it. I'm motivated to workout 30 more minutes for dessert. To me, it's like saving up—similar to not buying coffee for every weekday morning and getting a great new book each week instead. By working off those calories, I'm able to consume more calories in the delicious desserts that I love so much.

Skilled bakers, professional chefs, and chocolatiers are constantly creating irresistible pastries, hand-crafted truffles and delicious desserts! I love discovering new foods, especially sweet ones, so I'm always ready to fit in a workout in order to sample a new confection or innovative dessert.

Knowing myself and my propensity to go for everything new and delicious, I try to fit all my daily nutrients and vitamins in the smallest amount of healthy food I can. I aim to consume everything good that my body and mind need to get going, and still save room for the sweets I love! For more information on my savvy tips for integrating five food groups into meals and desserts, read *Got Sugar? Recipe Companion*.

To make a mental note of the healthy things you should be integrating into your diet, here's an updated, more accurate food pyramid. Keeping this in mind is just another game for me. I do my best to meet my body's healthy needs, but some days I need to carry-over my food choices to balance out other days later in the week!

Food Pyramid Guidelines

1 fat: This is a tough one. To keep it all balanced despite my sweets-intake, I keep active!

6-8 oz carbs: Sugary, bready, starchy, grainy things all fall under this category. For a benchmark amount, know that one slice of bread equals one ounce.

3 cups vegetables: So easy to integrate as a snack or into your meals.

2 cups fruits: Besides a great snack item, use them i breakfast recipes and desserts.

3 cups dairy: This usually equates to two glasses skim milk, one portion of yogurt or one portion of cheese.

5 oz protein: Focus on getting it through eggs, nuts and meat. If you're vegan, eating quinoa, sprouted seeds, soy foods or nuts with whole grains are also complete proteins. Think: one egg equals one ounce, two tablespoons of peanut butter equals one ounce, and a fist-sized portion of meat equals three ounces.

To my knowledge, it's best to eat a bit of protein with your carbs to minimize hormonal imbalance. To do this, try milk with cookies or eggs with toast, or simply exercise regularly. Blood sugar is in control when the two hormones (insulin and glucagon) in your blood are in balance. In response to eating carbohydrates, our pancreas produces **insulin**, the hormone responsible for storing fat or generating energy. On the other hand, both protein consumption and exercise produces **glucagon**, the hormone that promotes the activation and utilization of fat for energy. Check out glucagon on Britannica: http://www.britannica.com/EBchecked/topic/235785/glucagon, or other sources if interested in a more scientific explanation.

Also think about how you eat when you're not hungry. I do this occasionally, and I've wondered if it's some emotion propelling my decision to eat? Quite possibly if the desire to eat came when I was full, maybe I was happy, bored, frustrated or sad.

Since I run my business from home, food is readily available for instant comfort. When I get stuck writing, or become frustrated from a challenging photography portfolio, I've often headed for the bag of chocolate chips. I don't feel guilt, I just make a mental note about needing to exercise for two, not just one, reasons: to maintain my strength and health, and also to use up that extra fuel.

I might feel guilt when I get home at 9pm from a dinner out with friends and I realize how much I overate and drank socially from feeling happy. I still have to practice eating less of the gigantic portions that are served in most restaurants. But ladies, it's all a work in progress. We've got to eliminate the guilt and just move forward with finding a solution.

One way I do that is by knowing it takes a 3,500 reduction in calories to lose 1 pound. For me this equates to eliminating about 500 calories per day for 7 days. I like to split the amount and reduce my food intake by 250 calories for 6 days, and add 30 more minutes of workout for the other 250 calorie use, in order to avoid just eating 500 calories less per day.

I hate getting to this point, we all do. But when I get there, I move past the guilt and the problem, and commit to a healthy streak for a week. I write down food I've eaten on a notepad that I can leave for myself on the counter as a reminder. This helps me stay aware of the calories.

Keeping a food log definitely helps you realize your calorie intake. You might not realize how much you snack on your kids' foods! I know I didn't until I starting keeping a log. All of this comes back to the importance of knowledge. Be aware of how much and what you are eating. Be aware of slight weight gain, before it might get out of control. Know how to keep a food journal to constantly stay aware of your health and diet. Know how to keep that protein-and-carbs balance, in order to feel happy and avoid feeling lethargic.

Also, by staying aware of my food intake, it's like a game and my mind stays active: calculating, analyzing, and assessing my history and future strategies. This is essential so that I don't get too caught up in the results. Don't fret and sweat the big stuff, make a plan, use your brain, work toward that goal, and before you know it you'll be on your way in no time.

Yes, I wonder if I'll be able to meet my ideal end goal, but distracting myself from that large, looming goal ahead, which can be really daunting, with small attainable little goals is a great solution. I play little games with myself in order to reach those small goals and it helps me move along with an upbeat manor through each week.

With each small goal I've achieved, I feel rewarded. By letting go of that end goal, I don't let myself get down and frustrated if I don't lose the 3 pounds I was aiming to lose. *Just as important* as achieving the end goal is enjoying the attempts with small goals and games. Try to recognize all your mini-successes, so that whatever the outcome you'll feel positive and balanced. Know that you really did try your best and you won't get discouraged, annoyed or frustrated with trying it again.

Trigger Notes

After gaining some new knowledge, I may want to adopt a new strategy or system. To remind myself of this newfound discovery and plan, I tape reminder notes to my refrigerator and bathroom mirror. Taping reminders or trigger notes around are a great way to make sure your brain practices thinking in a new fashion. This way you're prompting your brain to form the habit or pattern that you want to develop.

Reading things once or absorbing knowledge once isn't enough to make a change. Continually reading and practicing healthy habits is how I make my healthy-shift stick. I read up on affirmations and learned they really do help. They really do promote positive change and positive mental attitude.

Notes that I've made in the past range from improving self-motivation and self-worth to simply remembering new habits. Here are a few that I've taped up, which have made a positive impact:

- Thoughts aren't real. Stress comes from believing in unnecessarily worrying thoughts.
- I am the perfect body for me.
- Make up a new game while doing a chore.
- Trust the phenomenon of life.
- Laugh at my brain—I don't ask it to create thoughts.
- Accept compliments. Give compliments.
- Life is filled with delightful surprises.
- Hug my kids four times a day.
- Believe in myself.
- I am lovable. I love.
- Stop eating the kids' leftover breakfast.

Basically, we all have behavior patterns that we use automatically to respond and react to our lives. Humans wouldn't have survived if we didn't learn what worked and what didn't. Since we need to be able to respond quickly to the environment and events around us, our brain references the past to make quick decisions. These are our learned responses and thought patterns. If some core behaviors, from which other responses are built, were formed in a situation not needed for today's survival, the "still" brain keeps referencing them. This makes it difficult to evolve into the mentally healthy direction that we aim for. By choosing to think optimistically and say positive affirmations, we will subconsciously refuse those outdated core behaviors and begin to reassess them. For me, affirmations worked! My mind realigned its thought processes by thinking about the statements more often, until they became an integral part of my lifestyle.

On the flip side, there's just so much to know! And health advice seems to change almost with every new generation of scientists. If I really think about it, scientists have their own set of behaviors and beliefs which color their research and results. So, in effect, the advice we cull is often subjective—you can't say that one piece of advice is the ultimate fact or the ultimate truth.

Almost as a contradiction to what I've tried to encourage you to think in terms of the importance of acquiring knowledge, I learned that it's just as important to give up knowledge. Be ready to reassess your thinking, your thoughts, that facts you thought you knew. After all there's always room for inight, as with everything in life.

By understanding and accepting that you'll never know the ultimate truths and mysteries about life, you'll be less confused. And by enjoying constant learning and editing that knowledge base, you'll be able to enjoy maintaining your fitness, health, and positive attitude. It's all part of the process. I feel better day-to-day armed with knowledge, as well as the understanding that it's very subjective and needs a grain of salt. In the end, I trust my intuition after all the knowledge I've accumulated.

Debunking Sugar Myths

Sugar has received a bad reputation over the years. But think: all carbohydrates including starches and sugars originating from foods like bread, peas, corn, pasta, fruit, candy bars are technically sugar, not just what's in your sugar bowl. Now, can all those things really be that bad? Let's reformulate our thoughts about sugar to get a more comprehensive understanding of what it is.

When consuming any carbohydrate, the digestive system breaks it down into simple sugars (glucose), which are carried through the bloodstream to nourish and energize cells. Whether or not it was from eating table sugar or a carrot, by the time it gets to the liver, it has been broken down to a glucose molecule. There's no way your body knows that the glucose molecule came from a carrot versus a grain of table sugar, except that the entire body benefits from more nutrients when consuming the carrot.

I've been scared by claims about how horrible sugar is to our bodies, so I began to research sugar online. The information is sometimes baffling and contradictory. Here are some thoughts on a few of the most intriguing, hot debates on sugar.

Myth: Sugar causes hyperactivity in children

I don't want to be the outcast mom, or be known as thoughtless when people see me allowing my kids to eat something sweet. So, I found many different studies from universities and clinics that concluded that there is little evidence that refined sugar plays a role in hyperactivity for most children.

1. Does Sugar Make Children Hyper?, by Robert Needleman, MD, FAAP, http:// www.drspock.com/article/ 0,1510,4126,00.html.

2. Another study published in the New England Journal of Medicine (http:// topics.abcnews.go.com/topic/New-England-Journal-of-Medicine)gave some kids sugared foods and others foods with artificial sweeteners. No notable difference was found.

3. Questions posed to the specialists at Cornell Center for Materials Research offered some more answers: http://

www.ccmr.cornell.edu/education/ask/
index.html?quid=241.

There seems to be no sugar rush. So why does it appear that kids get hyperactive when they eat too much candy? The affect is more likely from the caffeine. Caffeine is found in chocolate and some sodas and increases any person's energy.

Myth: Sugar causes cavities

I was really baffled by this, so I'm glad that I learned what's actually going on! Sugar can lead to tooth decay, so brush well and often. Floss, drink water or chew gum regularly after sweet treats, and cavities will less likely form.

But did you know sugar itself doesn't damage teeth? Several types of bacteria are present in the mouth that feed on sugar. When bacteria metabolizes sugar, it creates acids in the mouth which de-mineralize tooth enamel leading to decay.

Sugar at normal mealtimes does almost no harm to teeth because the exposure to sugar is not sustained and the other foods you eat tend to scrub your teeth clean of sugar. Fresh fruit is rarely a problem, even though it contains natural sugars, due to the cleansing effect of the fruit fibers.

Myth: Sugar consumption displaces other nutrients

Sugar is a relevant ingredient in many healthy foods. Several U.S. diet surveys showed that the consumption of sugar has little impact on vitamin and mineral intakes.

Vitamin and mineral consumptions are determined by the whole diet, not a single ingredient like sugar. That's why it is important to eat a variety of nutrient-rich foods. If people ate only corn, their diets would be deficient in most essential nutrients.

Myth: Sugar makes you fat

Sugar has only 15 calories per teaspoon and is no more fattening than any other 15 calories. Weight is gained by taking in more calories than your body burns for energy. Carbohydrates (like sugar, bread, fruit, and potatoes) and protein provide 4 calories per gram. Fats provide 9 calories per gram. One problem with sugars, however, is that many products add a high amount of sugar to sweeten the products. This, in turn, causes the product to be higher in calories. Because consuming more calories means you must expend more calories to reduce or manage your weight, this can be of concern.

Myth: Sugar causes diabetes

If you have diabetes, you do need to watch your sugar and carbohydrate intake to properly manage your blood sugar level. However, if you don't have diabetes, sugar intake won't cause you to develop the disease. The two main risk factors for Type 2 diabetes are being overweight and living an inactive lifestyle. Eating sweets does not cause diabetes. Inactive sugar lovers, however, may increase their chances of obesity, if more calories are consumed than burned each day. Inactivity and obesity are associated with people developing Type 2 diabetes.

Positive Habits

I've definitely aspired to integrate many positive habits, like practicing self-acceptance and demonstrating unconditional love and patience with my kids. But who am I kidding!

I can't actively and simultaneously maintain all the ideal positive traits and healthy habits that I dream of having. I have to admit, when I do succeed at maintaining a healthy diet, daily workouts and professional goals, I feel rushes of adrenaline, pride, and self-worth, which as you know feels incredible. But I can't keep that up year in and year out. So in order to continue being positive even though not hitting super-woman status on a weekly, daily, hourly basis, I need some more manageable expectations that I'm a allowed to meet, and I need some time off on ditching the food pyramid.

It's my constant goal to be aware of and monitor my moods, actions, and reactions to see when I feel best, though I may not perfect them daily. Food awareness as well as goal setting and game playing are fairly regular positive habits that I maintain for myself. And to keep myself balanced and happy, there is one positive habit that I stick to without fail: my daily exercise habit.

Everyone needs a primary positive habit as well as other positive habits that you're keeping up fairly regularly. You can't be super perfect as you may plan, but you can set goals and do your best to achieve them.

For me, daily exercise is the number one, primary positive habit that I maintain in order to feel great. Without the routine of daily exercise, I feel less happy. Endorphins don't flood my system and I lose momentum. I feel healthier, if I'm strong. As a result of my commitment to my positive habit, my confidence is boosted too. This then fuels a positive cycle. When I'm confident, I feel proud of myself, I'm positive throughout my day and I'm a better mom.

I haven't always been this habitual about exercise. After college, I wasn't biking to class every day and bopping around campus. I noticed I felt kind of melancholy and weak after a day of work in an office. In order to stop this state of being, I needed a change. So I decided to establish a new pattern of activity.

Almost 20 years ago, I started jogging and biking daily and started logging my feelings. I logged the exercise and hours in my day planner and assessed my state of being at the end of each week. Since then, I've trained myself that I must exercise for mental and physical well being, no matter what! It's a positive lifestyle habit. This habit has helped me eliminate wasting time and brain space on deciding whether to work out or not

—I just do. No thought needed, no questions asked. I simply wake up and I know I'm going to exercise (unless it's my one day off that week) and I know that I'll reap the benefits of a happy heart, positive mind, and healthy body (unless it's my one day off that week.)

Like most women, I've been through a lot in my life—getting a divorce, having best friends move away, losing relatives and dealing with job changes, not to mention changing hormones while needing to maintain composure through serious adult responsibilities. All these instances, that could present a lot of stress in life, needed to be balanced out with some positivity. This cemented even more the importance of exercise for me.

No matter how I ate, which job I had or didn't have, how poorly I reacted to my kids temper tantrums, or how I dealt with the newest crisis, I knew I would exercise and this would help me feel better. Knowing that I have one positive habit, knowing that I plan to achieve something, knowing that I'll do something good for myself no matter the troubles I face—this has surely saved me.

So, aside from needing exercise to balance out being highly interested in sugary things, it has helped me keep my confidence. I have stayed strong physically even when personal disasters have mentally paralyzed me.

Enjoy Everyday Life

Positive habits can help our perspective on life be one of enjoyment instead of annoyance. Beyond having a primary positive habit that grounds you in moving forward, other ones can be imbued throughout your daily life. For instance: try making chores a positive experience. Something simple like grocery shopping gives me joy.

I find product placement intriguing. I used to work in marketing so I love thinking about product designs, logos and where items are placed on the shelves. Some pay to be placed on prime shelves, some don't. I can relate to those smaller companies, since I'm also a small fish in the pond in terms of my own business and profession. So, out of empathy, curiosity, and if not solidarity, I support those small guys by buying products from their off-beat brands. Small habits like this make me happy and reinforce positivity.

I also stay positive by being organized at home. To stay organized, I keep a list of kitchen staples that I need to keep mealtimes going for my family. Each week I'll note the kitchen staples missing in my fridge or cupboards, and I'll use this once a week for a few meals (see 'Kitchen Staples' in *Got Sugar? Recipe Companion*). This means I'll spend less time on grocery shopping. Less time grocery shopping means I'll get more free time to fit in a workout. This is another game I play—I set a limited shopping time as a goal, and when I achieve it, I'm rewarded with more free moments. Another great aspect of this way of shopping is that with a steady flow of set choices, I get to engage more of my creativity. Say you only have cans of beans, tuna, black olives, and artichokes. Not sure what you could make out of it? I'll say, 'There's my sandwich!' I'll just mix it up with olive oil and put it on some whole grain bread.

You might wonder why this cognitive re-structuring and habit building doesn't work for diminishing my sweet tooth. It can. But I just love eating sweets—they make me feel giddy. I love savoring all the flavors and emotions that come with eating sweets. I simply enjoy making a game out of organizing my time to create them and equally enjoy staying active in order to earn them.

I appreciate all the artisan bakers, pastry chefs, chocolatiers and candy makers out there. I also love to bake. Creating a dessert brings happiness to my friends and family who enjoy the ritual of my offering! I won't lie, it makes me feel good to see others enjoying what I've made. I don't want to give up the joy I feel when creating or consuming a perfect balance of sweetness and texture. For me, this pleasure transcends so many different levels and aspects of my life that I've just taken it on as a part of my life. And really my healthy attitude is not mutually exclusive. I've made them work together and dovetail nicely so that one simply complements the other.

If I want to eat two delicious pastries for breakfast, an ice cream shake for lunch and have wine with dinner, I can do just that! Ok, I'll have gotten little if any nutrients, calcium or fiber. So to make this day nutritionally balanced, I'll drink 9 glasses of water throughout the day, take all my vitamins, and eat three prunes for fiber. I'll feel great having got all my nutrition, and happy to have enjoyed such luxurious treats as well. This would make me all the more motivated to do a great workout the next day!

Most days I enjoy trying to burn sugar off! I play a game, like an arcade game in my mind—and try to use up the calories I've put in. If I have to exercise 30 more minutes to use up that 300 calorie brownie sundae I ate, then so be it. I wake up 30 minutes

earlier and zap it out as energy expended,
remembering how I enjoyed my decision to eat it.

Big-Picture Goals

In order to do it all—gain and adopt new knowledge,
create positive habits, and make the most out of daily
life—you should create some big picture goals. My
main picture goals are:

1. Schedule time for daily exercise.
2. Be mindful of diet and calorie intake to
   maximize enjoyment of sweets.
3. Keep creating and learning lifestyle tricks, and
   playing games to increase metabolism, pride
   and self amusement.

Exercise Induces Positivity

Studies have shown that exercise brings about
significant increases in confidence and self-esteem.
Both aerobic exercise and resistance exercise suppress
appetite hormones and postpones hunger for about
two hours. Whenever I don't exercise, I'm hungrier and
more likely to fall victim to snacking. I'm here to
reassure you that you can stay fit and consume sugar

within reason. Doing it both is definitely feasible. Don't feel guilty, simply embrace it: be happy and do both!

Now, we know that exercise releases the hormone glucagon which helps offset insulin levels, which in turn helps you avoid an energy crash and stay physically pumped. Also, I find that exercise helps me cope and combat mental exhaustion. Mental exhaustion and physical exhaustion are two different things for me. When I am mentally beat, I find that doing 10 minutes of yoga, my night time circuit or walking the dogs really revives my energy level (read '15-minute Night Circuit' on page 37 for more). But don't take my word for it, try it out yourself! Physical exertion seems to actually help my mental fatigue!

Many times I'm mentally exhausted from meeting client deadlines, staying up late as I edit photos until 2 am, and sleeping less. Getting up at 6 am to walk the dogs and then working out before my kids rise for their school day at 7 am is challenging to say the least. But, every time I dare myself to resist the urge to snooze, I'm rewarded with pride. On top that, it gets easier each year!

Having a plan for exercise really does make all the difference for me! Here's how I stay on top of my exercise schedule:

- **Plan my week of exercise.** Each Sunday evening, I take 10 minutes to plan the following week. If exact times are written on the calendar, I don't back out. It's no longer about whether or not I'll do it. I will get the exercise in because it's planned. Even though I have a flexible schedule being a photographer, I also volunteer, coach, and write during the day. So in order to get my exercise into my busy daily schedule, I usually exercise first thing in the morning.

- **Keep the calendar visible.** I used to have it on the kitchen counter, but then my counter became cluttered. So, I bought a giant 24 inch x 36 inch entire year plastic calendar. I use a dry erase pen, can see the big picture of my year and absolutely love it. I map out short and long term plans (and write down the date of the event I'll do, as my training goal.)

- **Exercise with a friend.** Often I find that exercising with a friend can be entertaining: whether it's keeping each other company as we take bathroom breaks or joking about the exercise video we're doing. I was a solo runner and biker for years and being accountable to someone else is a great motivator. The soccer and softball teams that I coach hold me responsible for keeping active and fit. My healthy schedule is important to others—I feel needed, and feeling needed really feels great!

When I first started running with another marathoner, I learned that exercise buddies are invaluable for turning sessions of grueling training into fond memories. She was as beautiful a girl as any I'd ever befriended-sporting gorgeous teeth, skin, nails, makeup and hair. She wore pearls and beautiful clothing and kept her home and car immaculate. Within a month of running two to three times a week we were hacking, spitting, snorting, and farmer-johning side by side. The second month as the runs got longer, we were even relieving ourselves in random places. The silly times we shared definitely made those training sessions more enjoyable, especially because I didn't think of her as a hacker, spitter or road-side reliever!

- **Exercise early.** Although the thought of running at 6 am in the dark used to scare me, I have been rewarded a thousand fold with all the gorgeous sunrises, misty, ethereal landscapes and traffic-free routes. I've enjoyed the reward so much that I now actually prefer to exercise early. It gets it out of the way, so I don't have to schedule it in or think about it later. I occasionally swim with a masters swim team from 5:30 am to 6:30 am. It's awesome to see the sunrise around me as I turn to breathe, and being around other active men and women ages 21-60 is great energy to start off the day! It raises metabolism and I gotta say, I do feel peppier all day. British research found that cyclists could hold a harder pace for longer at 6:45 in the morning than at 6:45 at night. You have a store of energy that you can fully utilize before its get tapped into by all your other daily activities. Besides being more energized in the morning, the exercise will give you more strength and motivation for the rest of the day.

- **Find a happy place.** Since music inspires me immensely, I enjoy downloading it and making new playlists each month. When it comes time for my workout, I look forward to putting my earbuds in and taking off into another reality!

- **Pat yourself on the back.** Keeping a mental journal works for my motivation. But a good friend of mine takes note of her successfully completed workouts on a calendar with little symbols that work for her. She'll note '3R' for when a completed 3-mile run, or 'L' for a completed session of lifting. At the end of the week we're eager to reflect on our accomplishments by reviewing our physical efforts all week long, especially if we've indulged over the weekend!

Keep Reading

Aside from reading fitness and health magazines when I'm in the bathroom (that's where I stack them up), I read each night to inspire myself as well as relax. Even if it's just a single page, I'll get some reading in. There are three books on my nightstand at all times; two books relating to personal growth and one fiction.

For 15 years, I've been an avid reader of self-help, inspirational books. In my late 20s I went through a period where I was overworked at a corporate job, then moved away from all my family and friends to open my own business in a new town, which was stressful. But by jumping into life opportunities, I got to know myself.

Through these difficult life changes, I learned techniques to feel accepting and loving of my abilities to make choices, and to lighten up in order to enjoy what I used to think of as stress. By reading great advice, I learned to create a peaceful inner state of being, one which brings me fulfillment that's completely independent of my external environment—whether it's calm or torrential, I'm centered, balanced and peaceful. This has been a continuous and integral part of my life.

Beyond reading about mental, emotional and inner well-being, I read about physical well-being. By reading up on physiology, I'm on track to stay healthy and active. It's during quiet reading times that I'm reminded that counting calories and portions are just games my mind plays. I don't need to get too serious about record keeping. Just have fun being aware of all aspects of health (including nutritional content and calories) and be aware of how the mind can interpret those things. Sometimes, the mind gets carried away with information, and might start obsessing over a single detail, fact, or goal. That's not healthy so let it go, stay aware and keep moving forward. Usually I laugh at what bubbles up in my mind, realize it's the mind's job to solve problems (imaginary or real) and continue to read inspirational books to further develop my happy, healthy mind.

There is so much interesting information just waiting to be harvested and taken on board. It feels great to continually educate and improve myself with this information! But after awhile of reading philosophy and personal growth books, I need to dive into fiction.

Reading fiction, on the other hand, is equally important. Fiction sweeps me into another reality, pulling me away from my daily duties, plans, thoughts, and worries. In this way it calms me. Fiction also exposes me to a new experience, a new way of seeing something, a new place, a new culture. This fresh, different take on life, helps keep me on my toes so that I integrate new positive ways of looking at the world and my life.

Realize Positive Intent

Life is like a great movie. All people are characters in it and they are probably doing what they think is the best decision. I know I'm doing what I believe is positive for myself and the world. Sure, I feel mad, disappointed or annoyed sometimes when things don't align exactly as planned. But I try to laugh at my reactions and smile at how passionate my feelings can be. I breathe in my aggravated feelings and acknowledge them. Then I let them go by immediately baking, reading a page in an inspirational book, cranking out 15 push ups or doing something in which I know I can excel. When I dissipate the negative feelings faster, I can get back to feeling proud and confident, which makes me even more determined to keep practicing my positive habits!

I jump in and open the door to whatever positive direction life is unveiling. I try my hardest, fight for what I believe in, and don't give up, but I've consciously developed a habit of letting go of whatever outcome. Sometimes life throws you hardships and sometimes you don't achieve your goal, but you've done your best and this is what counts.

I give my all to practicing positive habits and working towards maintaining a fun, active, encouraging, balanced, happy lifestyle. That's all anyone can do, right? I've spent 10 years practicing this concept of believing—that with a small seed you can develop positive intent.

Life offers so many possibilities and it's no fun to be stalled by the fear of the result being sub-par or not what you expected. By believing that whatever result *is the right one*, I'm able to leap into more adventures and enter more discussions because I believe every action leads to the right outcome. In this way, I'm constantly trying and learning new things. This gives me an open mind, and with an open mind, I am less judgmental since I've seen many ways work for the better.

I'm reminded of a Chinese story called "Good Luck, Bad Luck!" where things that seem like bad luck (their horse runs away) turn out to be good luck (when it returns with a herd of horses.) And how good luck (new wild horses) turns out to be unfavorable (the son breaks his leg trying to tame one) which leads to good luck (the son not being drafted when the army comes for abled-bodied youth.) My take away: don't try to judge anything. If I catch myself placing a "good/bad" label on things, I recognize it now, because for months I taped up the phrase "no good, no bad" on my bathroom mirror. By thinking this way, you can let go of feelings (easier) from your mate not noticing your needs, hearing people talk behind your back, not achieving a goal you set or not making that traffic signal because your mind takes it less personally. *Who knows* if it's good or bad luck - just keep acting with positive intent and believing that the outcomes are destined to be whatever they are based on your intent and other influences in life, and that's all you can do.

Healthy Sweet Tooth

A sugar-injected healthy diet is satisfying! I drink milk with my cookies. I add chopped spinach and walnuts to brownies. I make sweet treats with healthy items like fortified cereal. Knowing I'm getting something of nutritional value in my sweets makes me feel great.

Pulling together daily family dinners aren't always easy as pie. But I grew up enjoying the family meals we ate together at the table, so I want to keep this positive tradition going. For the most part I try to ride the line between fun and firm. I catch myself saying things like 'Get your elbows off the table' and 'Sit up straight, don't lay down next to your plate.' I also find myself wishing it was time for dessert.

After all, dessert puts everyone in a good mood. It always amazes me how well my kids behave when dessert is at stake. This is just one more reason to eat it every night!

At the dinner table with my kids, I try to ask a question or have a contest relating to health and sweets: 'Whoever finishes all their veggies first gets five chocolate chips', 'Does cake have any nutrition in it?', or 'Where does sugar come from?'

If I don't know the answer, the kids and I do some research. We'll look things up online or discuss the possible answers during our meal. These kinds of games at meal time are so successful because they engage the entire family. By the time we have dessert, we're functionably happy, having fun.

As a mother, just as in other arenas in life, I want to be playful and amusing as well as serious and knowledgeable. One without the other makes like too mundane.

> *"I learned that courage was*
> *not the absence of fear, but*
> *the triumph over it."*
> -Nelson Mandela

Challenge Fears

We're all creatures, living here on earth, afraid of a variety of things relating to our personal history. But the more times I face a fear and get past feeling anxious, the more I feel liberated. I'm having way more fun feeling uncomfortable and later elated by my attempts, than I was just settling for where I was and feeling regret and wonder.

Recognizing that I'll either feel fear (if I'm going to attempt something new or challenging) or regret, (if I choose not to engage in the opportunity) has led me to take on challenges more and feel the effects of fear. I prefer feeling uncomfortable from overcoming a fear, than feeling uncomfortable from regret or wondering if "I should have". This way I get to learn a lot of new things along the way of overcoming a fear, which expands my knowledge base of things possible on earth. Expanding knowledge leads to increased understanding and acceptance of the variety of ways people choose to live!

I have two school-aged kids and no employer. Managing my own business, I challenge fears and battle self-doubt daily. I must keep working hard and pursue my passions of photography and writing to earn this lifestyle I so enjoy.

I think the power of positive habits is kicking in here, since I'm writing the *Got Sugar?* series. I've thought of dozens of reasons why my books aren't needed in the world, that they're not unique enough, that the information's already out there. But since I'm practicing challenging my fears, I've kept at the mission, and here are the fruits of my work.

Same goes for exercise: Whether I'm taking a new class at the gym or attempting a faster pace than I think I can do, I just try it. I might try it for a short period of time and give myself an out-option if necessary—but at least I still go for it. Many times I'll just hang in there and end up surprising myself by doing better than I thought I would. If it turns out I'm less embarrassed than I thought I'd be, I feel proud in tackling something outside of my comfort zone.

When I started college, I had no waterskiing experience. A boyfriend taught me how to get up on one ski on our first spring break. Soon after, I joined the waterski team at University California of Santa Barbara. Seeing 18-20 year olds excel at waterskiing techniques and tricks was truly eye-opening! I leapt into a new, exciting world, a world of waterskiing, sport, and challenges. Discovering these sportswomen and sportsmen, discovering the sport, and discovering all that I could learn from waterskiing was truly amazing. I'd never known this community and these events even existed, until I gave it a try. Quickly I learned about ideal body-form for slalom courses, skiing tricks, and ramp-jumping. The more I was exposed to, the more I soaked up every experience. I learned how to master the different speeds of the boat for any event at waterski tournaments and practiced everything I was taught. I found it so rewarding to improve a skill. By my senior year, I knew how to drive a ski boat at various speeds and I competed against other colleges. This sport was one of the best parts of my college experience. By taking that first step and trying something new, I bonded and grew with 20 fun, smart, hard-working, water-loving people.

Fast forward to this year when I visited Park City, Utah for a reunion with my college roommates. Throughout the course of my college career, I had gained seven wonderful roommates. And now we get together annually for a long reunion weekend. We went to Olympic Park to watch the freestyle aerial skiers train for their jumps off long ramps into a huge swimming pool. This is how they practice with the lack of snow during the summer.

When entering a local museum on one our play-days, I spotted a sign that offered three-hour classes to the public. My heart skipped a beat as I excitedly decided to join. I signed up before I could talk myself out of paying $95. In no time, I was practicing jumps on the trampoline into the pool. Then with ski boots, skis, and a helmet on, the instructor pointed up the stairs I had to climb with the simple words, 'go for it!'

Standing at the top of the ramp, I thought, 'This is going to propel me straight up into the air.' This was something new, the jump was quite high. The thought of it was exhilarating and unbelievably scary all at once. I knew I just wanted to do it. So I let go, trusting the physics of the ramp and keeping my eyes level with the horizon. I flew down that ramp and jumped! The feeling of being airborne was like no other feeling.

By the end of three hours, I had accumulated a number of unsuccessful jumps and some really sore quads. But all in all, the experience was amazing and I had accomplished all three of my goals: complete a 360° helicopter move, a back flip, and a front flip.

Had I not joined the waterski team back in college, I wouldn't have launched off that wood ramp in Park City. Every person I've ever met, every book I've read, every experience I've participated in, every time I actively listen, I'm rewarded for challenging my fears, whether immediately or later in life. Each attempt opens doors that wouldn't have opened.

Beyond physical activities, stepping outside your comfort zone in your relationships at work or at home is also important. Discussing money issues with roommates, talking about hurt feelings between family members, or confronting parents or coaches regarding fairness in sports can definitely stretch limits and prompt awkwardness. When addressing whatever problem at hand, I try hard to view myself as a character in a movie, and wonder how the awkwardness will turn out. After all, these little bumps keep me interested in life.

So with any difficult challenge, whether physical, work related or emotional, the best motto truly is Nike's: just do it.

"Leap and the net will appear."

-A Zen saying

Don't Worry, Be Curious!

There are probably hundreds of ways to diet and lots of different books and articles on strict no-sugar diets, fasting diets, no-dairy diets and cookie diets. You name it, it's all been written.

Since I like to keep myself amused and entertained with life's routine activities, I've tried many styles of dieting and working out. I don't worry. I'll just try it because it's different and because I'm curious.

I am intrigued by the creativity behind these different diets! Don't beat yourself up with worries if the new diet you want to dabble in doesn't work out. Obtaining knowledge through a variety of sources and trusting feelings of well-being is all a person can do. Experimenting will help figure out what feels the best!

For awhile I tried the no-carb diet. I ate as little as two slices of turkey for breakfast, tuna on a bed of lettuce for lunch and normal dinner. I felt remarkably full for how little I'd eaten. Several weeks passed and then I realized, 'I liked my life with sweets, I'm not this rigid.' I like baking and feeling like a kitchen scientist! I know myself better and have chosen to compensate in other ways to stay strong and healthy to make my life work for me.

Get Sugar!

Sugar comes in a variety of forms. Yes, in the edible form, but also in the form of love! I receive sugar from my friends and family and am endlessly smitten and utterly grateful. I give and get sugar from my kids with their loving hugs and their desire to play with me! In my home, we like to say, 'Gimme some sugar!' or 'Who wants some sugar?' as we spread the love! Finding ways to give and receive sugar in the form of love makes life sweeter yet. And I find that sugar always results in me getting some sugar in return!

When my son hit the end of 2nd grade, he stopped responding to my over-zealous good-bye hugs and professions of love for him at drop-off. I felt the you're-embarrassing-me vibe. So, we made up a game so he doesn't have to say 'I love you' in public. We agreed that when I drop him off curbside at his grammar school we would look into each other's eyes, hold it for 1 second and smile big as we say yelled, 'Byyyyyyyyye!' As long as I have something that equates to an 'I love you, mom!', I'm good!

Another thing I'm increasingly aware of is how fast time goes by. If I don't plan a daily tradition with my kids, before I know it the day's gone and I've gotten no sugar-loving! All of a sudden it's time to make dinner, sit together for a meal, shower, read, and shove off to bed. Having seen many days end up like this, I started a ritual of making something together as soon as they got home from school. It ranges from peanut butter balls to pumpkin bread for my son, and from angel food cake to chocolate chip cookies for my daughter. Regardless of the result, we work together for 10-15 minutes creating something. After that I work in my office, as they complete homework assignments. As a reward for our dedicated effort we have a freshly made treat that we'll reconvene to consume!

I keep adding positive habits one at a time, as they relate to a need I have. The tradition above evolved because I needed to share more sugar, or love, with my kids. I needed more bonding time that didn't have a reason. We have to do homework, we have to go to practice, we have to do chores, etc. I wanted to create time together where we weren't just pulled together for some task. So, I sat and thought what I could do with both of them, in a short amount of time, which would create a lasting memory and give me a short-term love-fix. Cracking, mixing, melting, kneading, rolling, cutting in the kitchen works for me. For one of my college roommates and her kids, a board game or drawing time works. There's no right answer. There's just continual change as kids grow and my life develops. We just need to review the change and adapt to meet these new needs. Everything shapes me. That's why it's important to review the small things in life. These are small ways I can make myself happier while being responsible. If I'm not doing things to bring me joy through my chore-laden days, it's not shaping me or my family in the direction of more joy when the next changes happen.

I'm excited to see how I'll change my daily habits or traditions to fit my family's needs next year, then the next, and the next. I look forward to the challenge of adjusting to change and the heaps of sugar that will come.

Chapter Two:

Lifestyle Tips and Tricks

Fly like a hummingbird, darting lightly through each day, looking to experience the core sweetness of all people, places, things and situations of life.

Life gets mundane. Life gets busy. Life is serious. I'm a single mom and a professional photographer. My daily life requires a lot of planning, responsibility, and a great big heaping of level-headedness. Accomplishing my dreams—well, most of them—as an entrepreneur and a mother is what keeps me sane!

From the big things like volunteering at the grammar school or coaching my kids' sports teams, to the things that often go unnoticed like finding the best health insurance rates for my family or making sure my kids have clean underwear. With school functions, work, sports and the duties incorporated into home-life, my calendar is like a jigsaw puzzle.

While facing the responsibilities of adulthood can be draining, life can be entertaining when you embrace a child-like spirit.

As discussed before, one of the ways I stay upbeat is by practicing playfulness while accomplishing my goals. I set challenges and play games that remind me to sip the nectar in whatever situation. It's easy to get sucked through a blur of life by the fast-paced world.

To keep life light and keep myself entertained, I'll bring out my child-like spirit when doing the simplest things. When withdrawing money at an ATM, I'll distort my lips in funny ways for the camera. It's also great to think that I'm the only mom who does such crazy things to stay child-like. I need to laugh, or I find I'll start resenting my adulthood, wishing I didn't have to grow up to be in charge of so many things. Anyway, a simple thing like making funny faces makes banking much less of a chore, I'm a right?

I even get a kick out of my self-induced competitions that inspire me to move faster and make the most of my tight schedule. Some mini-competitions include clocking my dishwasher unloading time, and trying to beat the time each week. 'I am such a geek,' I think to myself often. Interestingly enough, the more often I embody the geek in me, the happier I am completing my tasks. The more meaningless games I come up with, the more fun games bubble up in my head without even trying, as I journey through life. And I get the added benefit of laughing at myself when I come up with some of the ridiculous games that I usually do.

I also think, 'Why not?!' I'll just try some new made-up game to see if it can be done. I also think, 'I wonder if anyone else has ever unloaded the dishwasher this fast, or on their tippy-toes, or with one eye-closed the whole time.' The whole process is silly and fun and that's the point. Injecting some of this light-hearted spirit is what keeps me balanced in the sea of routine, chores, and responsibility. When you make things silly and fun, it's no longer just a duty.

Just doing something amusing amuses me. When I do something creative, fun, silly, daring, joyous or uninhibited, I'm living in this moment. I'm focusing on having fun in the present, no matter if I have duties and chores. I'm having fun now, I'm laughing now, not later, not postponing it endlessly, not ever smiling and having a laugh because I never get around to it. This is what game playing is about for me—living for the now.

The more I do it, the more it happens naturally, and it becomes a positive habit.

My job affords me the flexibility to engage in these random lifestyle games I talk about in this chapter; after a photography shoot I can wait and edit photos after my kids' bedtime and do it until 2 am if I need to.

If you work 9-5, you won't be doing your work with one eye closed or nipping away to get your swim workout in during afternoon public lap times. But many of my habits can be incorporated to some extent, however infrequent. Try them out at home, make yourself laugh at your desk, share a silly moment with your coworkers.

Time-savers

The main thing I need is more time. I need more time to do all the things I have to do, all the things I'm curious to try, all the things that I want to do as a loving parent. So first thing's first, find time to do everything, and then you can find your way of incorporating the fun.

Here are some things that I do to free up time for baking, my family tradition, and exercising, my main positive habit:

- **Buy ice cube trays**: Use these as jewelry organizers. Two will stack on top of each other in the drawer. Annoying, time-wasting searches for earring pairs has become a thing of the past!
- **Learn computer commands**: Every time I open or close a window, or copy and paste text, I look at the shortcut commands next to its name in the pull-down menu. Now, I do Command+C for Macs or Ctrl+C for PCs, in order to copy (and countless other commands)instead of dragging my cursor up to the menu bar and clicking around. This saves me precious minutes.
- **Shop on-line:** I do this occasionally to save time. Instead of driving, parking and getting sidetracked by cool sale items, shopping online is direct and quick. I keep a notepad by my phone and wait to gather a group of items for one order. Many web sites offer free shipping over $50. I shop at local stores to support them as much as possible too.
- **Play games to move faster**: I time myself when grabbing a jacket for my kids who are

already buckled in and then suddenly realize they forgot to grab it for school. I time myself when unloading the dishwasher or washing machine. The kids have fun timing me, making me sprint. I lunge and dart around to beat the last time. I do this with a smile and my kids think I'm fun. I get the chores done faster and have more free time to exercise. I'm telling you it's a win-win situation.

- **Exercise two days a week at home**: For me, this saves me 20 minutes driving time R/T.

- **Brush my teeth in a different area of my house each day**: This one's pretty creative! While brushing with my right hand, I walk around and organize stuff with my left hand. I'll tidy all my medicine in a cabinet, I'll throw out expired stuff. As I'm brushing I'll tackle the kids' bathroom, I'll change the dirty washcloths, throw out the old toothpaste, and wipe off their counter. Super time-saver!

- **Use canned beans and frozen veggies**: For everything from soups and chilis to main meals and side dishes, these will save you from loads of prep time. No need for washing and cutting, simply plop them in and you're ready to go.

- **Type a list of birthdays and important events, and buy cards in advance:** While waiting at a car wash or other random time-zapping errands, I'll grab these cards so that I don't have to go out to buy them at the last minute in the future. It feels great to be organized, and when it comes time for someone's birthday, I'm thrilled and proud of how prepared I was!

- **Eat energy bars for lunch.** When traveling or errand running, I always pack an energy bar: I substitute it for lunch. Doing so gives me more time for sightseeing and walking around or errand-running since I won't have to sit and wait at a restaurant! And since other cities and countries have unusual, unique desserts, I always want to save some room for trying these out. By eating an energy bar for one of my meals, I'll have more room for dessert!

- **Group errands or chores:** When I drive out of my small town to the nearest Mac Superstore, I plan to swim laps during the window of available public times, hit Costco, buy any known family birthday present needed in the next month, and grab pet supplies. Bi-weekly I need crickets for my tree frogs' diet. I've been known to strategize my errand runs so well, that I don't ever backtrack as I loop around town. If the pet store is open, earliest, I'll hit them first, then Costco, which opens next. Then I take my ventilated plastic carrying case full of

30 crickets into the pool locker room, since the car is too hot in the sun. They'll chirp and sing for an hour for showering and changing women —how cute is that!

Perfecting Music Playlists

Musicians are my heroes. Their ingenuity of beats and lyrics continually inspire me. Since I like doing things to the beat of music, I make different playlists for each type of workout. After years and years of working-out daily, I need a constantly updated variety of music to stay fired up.

In order to find out what song will work best for a certain type of activity you need to figure out a song's BPM (beats per minute). To figure out a song's BPM, count the beats in 10 seconds of the song and multiply it by 6. If you count 20 beats in 10 seconds, then multiply 20 beats by 6 to get 120 BPM.

Weights Playlist

Test out your lifting pace to see what beat you enjoy most. Take biceps for example: I lift up for two beats and down for two beats. This works out to 120 BPM, so

I would choose a song with that BPM like Phil Collins'
Sussudio.

Aerobic Activity Playlists

Steady or Mellow Pace
Feel the beat of a song for a more relaxed aerobic
workout. When your foot hits the ground, or pedal
goes around, find a song to match your pace. For me,
80-82 BPM matches my pace for steady runs or
cycling. Nickelback's *Someday* is a good example of a
song with 80 BPM.

Speedier Pace
Interval training (an intense burst of speed followed by
an easy pace) is an important aspect of muscle
conditioning. Having songs to match that faster pace
makes it more enjoyable; it helps me focus on trying to
stay with the beat. Lily Allen's *Smile* is a good one with
96 BPM.

Push-It Pace
Once you know the BPM that you comfortably run at,
let's just say 70 BPM, go find three songs at that
mellow pace. Then find another three at a pace slightly
higher, like 75-80 BPM. Arrange them in an alternating
pattern, so that you get a push-it song after your

mellow song. This way, every other song pushes you to run a tad faster than your normal pace.

To keep up with a faster beat, make your steps shorter; don't take big strides, little shuffles are good, just hit the beat. If you'd like to test a push-it pace, try Black Eyed Peas *Pump It* which has 77 BPM. Even if you don't like the song, you'll be able to hear the beat easily.

Being in the car with the radio turned on is tons more fun when trying to distinguish a song's BPM. While driving, I listen and count out the BPM of new songs to go home and download.

> *"The quickest way to become an old is to stop learning new tricks."*
> -John Rooney

Everything's a Game!

Creating positive habits, for no other reason than to entertain, induces more interesting results! Life is an adventure, professionally and personally, and I try to recognize and jump into the adventure every day!

When I started playing games to amuse myself, I never would have guessed it would have evolved into such a mini-goal-oriented-daily-fun habit. But I found that the more challenges or goals I created, no matter how incidental, the more feelings of pride surfaced. If I won or succeeded, I would be happy and not bogged down with all the responsibilities bestowed upon us with adulthood. In order to achieve many of my goals professionally, I've had to reach out and ask for help. This scares me, so I stand up whenever I make nerve-racking phone calls to new or distant friends when networking and searching for advice. Standing up and pacing a certain spot in my house sounds silly, but knowing it's my game, gives me comfort. Now the game has changed to see if I can stop pacing within 3 minutes, down from 5 minutes earlier this year.

Exercising for 30 minutes a day in itself is a great game. But taking it easy the other 23 hours and 30 minutes doesn't give me energy or strength and it doesn't help me burn off the sweets that I love. So, I began to view every activity or chore as a game. By doing 30 seconds here, a minute there, it helps make my life way more entertaining; I amuse myself and my kids. Because I act like a kid daily through these games, I also feel less annoyed about being an accountable adult weighed down with chores and responsibilities.

Another thing I think about when consciously choosing to run around, is how Native Americans must have lived, always active, hunting, and gathering. Life was more physical in the past, and for people today our lives are centered on a lot of sitting in offices. I sit a lot for work, I sit while writing, I sit while editing photos. This is not active. So I make sure I exercise through playing these games. I have a lot of fun trying to simulate the life of an active hunter or gatherer in my little games.

Yosemite always reminds me of what life must have been like before the turn of the century. I can't imagine being an early settler in the winter. They must have had to keep moving just to stay warm! Hiking with my kids, I found myself curiously watching the time it took us to hike half a mile uphill at a normal pace. Then we figured out the half-way mark on the map and guessed our arrival time, selected a lunch break spot, and estimated the total time for our 7-mile hike.

This may seem like no big deal, but having the big picture in mind kept morale boosted. These goals, though inadvertent, gave us something to talk about as we hiked. We stopped many times to enjoy the views, gather sticks, and dip our toes in the river's edge. We guessed several times how long various lengths of our journey would take. How long would it take to get up to that ridge? Could we make up for lost time if we'd spent time gazing at waterfalls? Besides witnessing the obvious beauty of Yosemite Valley, we felt elated by our accomplishment. The light-hearted spirit and our mini-goals helped make the 6-hour uphill playful and enjoyable.

Active Games

- **Digging holes**, boogie boarding and collecting shells and sticks. I do whatever my kids do at the beach. The trick is to keep up with the kids' pace!
- **Sliding** with socks on my hardwood floors as I run between rooms. Remember, *Footloose*?! Yeah, you do! Let that inner rock-star in you free!
- **Trotting with the shopping cart and hopping onto the foot bar** as you go from the farther end of the parking lot to the store entrance. It's entertaining to see other shoppers have a double take as an adult glides by on a shopping cart.

- **Focusing on foot speed**. Trot upstairs using every step. Next time trot up stairs skipping a step. Time which one was faster. When my kids are loaded in the car off to school and yell, 'Mom, I forgot a jacket,' I can bound upstairs without wondering how much time I need. I know because I timed myself already! Oh, yes! I feel awesome when I get that jacket in as little time as humanly possible. And in the near future I'll be timing them! But currently, since they're not seasoned fast-jacket-retrieval sprinters, I'll play the game myself.
- **Playing hide and seek.** Tip-toe silently and slowly for 10 minutes as the finder. This engages leg and core muscles as you do so. Surprising the kids when you find them is good clean fun!

Chore-related Games

- **Washing dishes on my tippy-toes** without falling. After 10 minutes of it, spinning and lunging occasionally for interest, your calves will feel it and your heart rate will be elevated!
- **Unloading dishes or laundry using only one arm** for one minute. Then only the other arm for a minute.

- **Loading the dishwasher one item at a time** really fast to engage my abs. Grab each item from the sink, turning fast with a tight core to load the machine, then reach back to the sink, and repeat. This means that I leave dishes in the sink for the whole day, just so I can play this game with as many items available for a full two minutes for maximum abdominal action!

- **Folding two baskets of laundry before the next commercial break** or timing myself as I fold a load of laundry. I can try to beat it next time.

- **Bicep-curling with grocery bags** as I carry loads into the house. Or I just might see if I can carry all the bags in one trip to test the superhero strength of my upper body!

- **Picking up the pace** when raking leaves, doing light housework or gardening. Grab tools quicker, move faster and have fun trying to do chores faster than normal.

- **Making organization a game.** I challenge myself and my kids to find the most matching socks in the laundry pile, or to set the table in under a minute. We'll try to add different goals to the chores next time to keep us entertained.

- **Collecting doggie-doo.** Buy clear plastic gloves at the dollar store, in packs of 100, and kids will get a kick out of wearing them for picking up doggie-doo. *Make a game*: whoever collects the most poop in their trash bag wins "relax time" and gets out of the next chore...setting the dinner table.

Lifestyle Tips

- **Rewards for efforts.** Every day I hear myself tell my kids 'If you finish your homework by 4pm and do all your chores, you'll earn a reward.' Now I apply the same theory to myself! The main reward for me is feeling proud, which is timeless, and my kids seem proud to have a strong mom who can set up and take down our campsite single-handedly. But sometimes that just might not be enough, so having a back-up reward like a brownie sundae truly does the trick!
- **Get up and stand up.** I get up from my chair each hour, as I work. I'll go to the farthest bathroom, deliver a message by hand instead of emailing or run outgoing mail to an official blue mail box instead of using the red flag on my mailbox. If you need motivation to do this: a bowl of M&Ms in another room helps me get up

from my office more often, with an allotted five M&M's per visit.

- **Practice good posture.** I envision having a malt ball or pile of cotton candy on top of my head that I must keep from falling! Other times I stand up tall and pretend there is a balloon on a string tied to my rib cage up through my neck and out the top of my head.
- **Keep house temperature cooler**. It saves money, conserves energy, and keeps me moving to stay warm. My thermostat is set to 62° F.
- **Shop for exercise gear.** Exercising provides mental happiness, and shopping for gear makes me excited to be up on the latest trends. Good gear makes me want to wear it to get out!
- **Get a dog.** Even on blustery days, my two dogs need to get out. In terrible weather, without dogs, I would never go out. But getting out in strange weather is beautiful. You get to see things like ethereal mist, beautiful wind, and crisp cold. A beautiful way to take a quick, healthy break!
- **Subscribe to a fitness magazine**. I leave them by every toilet and flip through them when sitting in the bathroom. I'm always reminded to try a new exercise or a new recipe. It's also easier to take in one bite of information

at a time, as opposed to reading and trying to internalize an entire magazine all in one go.

- **Bookmark websites and blogs that educate and inspire you.** Here are a few of mine:

  www.goalsfortheweek.com
  A stay-at-home mom sets weekly goals for her different life roles and takes on triathlons.

  www.Hungry-Girl.com
  A blog that showcases and reviews the newest, tasty low-cal foods.

  www.Eatbetteramerica.com
  A great collection of easy recipes.

- **Perform actions of strength.** For example, I'll go camping for only one night which requires a lot of physical strength to set up and take down the tent and gear quickly! In another example, on a smaller scale, I pull my stomach in really tight as I refill ice cube trays with my purified water dispenser and as I carry them to the freezer. Doing things like that all day, engage my muscles and help me use what I consume! I want that cookie after dinner!

- **Race to and from places.** My kids love to play this with me. The airport is a great place for this. We race to the moving platforms, one of us hops on, and then the others see if we can beat the one on the platform to the end. This way we're active before sitting for a long period. We also run from the trampoline to the sink to wash hands before dinner.

- **Start small and follow through.** When I find myself annoyed at a chore, I come up with a game to push me through it or a reward for trying, and attack one chore at a time. When choosing the sock drawer to on focus, if I do extra sorting like underwear and bras, I'll get a bonus pat on the back. When I set expectations low in some situations, I'll get to meet and exceed them!

Diet Tips

- **Energy bars on-hand in two places: the car and my purse**. I always have a backup so I don't start opening boxes of cookies at the grocery store. Although, I still might be guilty of that!
- **Eat protein at every meal.** Protein keeps me fuller for longer. So when it comes time for sweets, I don't gorge!
- **Leave a full glass of water out** on the counter or desk, so it's ready to drink.
- **Split dinner** with a friend and save room for dessert.

- **Hard boil 6 eggs once a week.** They're the easiest source of all essential amino acids in the egg white.
- **Suppress hunger or boredom with exercise and water.** Next time a hunger pain surfaces, drink a glass or water and do three minutes of movement like marching in place, moving arms in big circles, doing 120 sit-ups, or running up three flights of stairs. Then wait 15 minutes. If still hungry after that, then eat! If the feeling passed then maybe it was at an unnecessary habitual time that could be broken. Every month I seem to have to play this game to retrain my mind's response to my stomach's misfired cue, to match my caloric needs.
- **Chew gum.** Gas stations make me smile, because while the gas is pumping, I get to check out the latest gum flavors! I'll have great breath and clean my teeth in between sweets.
- **Fast.** Seasonally, for just one day, I drink water, tea, and vegetable juice. It makes me feel lighter and it jump starts my short-lived healthy streak.
- **Make exceptions every week.** For example, I adjust food intake. I'll only eat a small, high-protein breakfast, skip lunch, and forgo snacks, if I know I'm going out for wine, salad, a full dinner and dessert later that evening!

- **Don't deprive.** Usually, when I deny myself what I'm craving, I end up eating it anyways, so sometimes I just skip a meal and enjoy whatever it is I'm craving. If I only eat an amazing piece of homemade cake for dinner, I make sure to take vitamins and exercise.
- **Track calories.** I approximate that running for 10 minutes burns 100 calories, and that walking for 10 minutes burns 50 calories. I log my time spent walking and running. I also keep a mental log of the obvious sugar and alcoholic indulgences. I try to match the exercise that same day or first thing the next morning to use any stored sugar as fuel!

Fitness Tips

- **Leave running shoes (and swimsuit for me) in the car, and music player in purse.** Occasionally I'll pull over when driving and run 20 minutes out and back. This is always refreshing to see the different neighborhoods and landscapes. It's like eye candy!
- **Keep a gym class or pool lap time schedule** in car glove box. Whenever I'm out I'll try fit in a workout, especially since I already have shoes and suit in the car at all times. In case I have unexpected errands come up and need to run

out, and forget to check the schedule before I leave home, I can make sure I don't miss an opportunity by being able to check the schedule while I'm already out.

- **Keep all workout clothes in one drawer.** Socks, bras, shorts, shirts, bands, hats, workout plans or books to reference. One spot makes it super easy to get ready without wasting a second of your day! In the morning, when making breakfast, I can run from the kitchen to the bedroom, get dressed, remind myself of the workout I want to do, and return to open the waffle maker.

- **Lay out gym clothes the night before**. If it's in plain view, I'll use it right away.

- **Change up the exercise.** Instead of just walking or running steady, I add skipping, side steps, or trotting backwards for 40 seconds, about six to eight different times into my run. I'll do my weight workout in reverse order or look up a new exercise for triceps and change the move in the workout. This keeps things fresh and interesting.

- **Write down exact time.** If I haven't made an exact start and end time, it doesn't motivate me to do it. I can find a million things to do *that need to be done*, so I need a start time. On Sunday nights, I write down the times of a daily workout schedule directly onto my calendar for each day.

- **Sign up for one exercise event each year.** Events make me more excited to exercise. Just one event a year keeps me thinking of the reason to maintain my strength. I enter a running race every year. So, sign up for a 5k race. Go ahead and try it. Search 5k races online, right now. Put the book down and challenge your fears! You can walk fast instead of run. Or you can run a quarter mile then walk another quarter mile, and continue in shifts through the whole race! Each race is always a fundraiser for something. By paying the entry fee you can feel good about donating! A race will also give you a good reason to go buy some cool new shorts! The power you get when training for something is unbelievable—it's great motivation!

- **Watch active people** on TV when working out. Program your DVR, TIVO, or MOXIE BOX to record shows that are fun, active and inspiring! My favorites are Wipeout, Minute to Win It, Survivor, Amazing Race, So You Think You Can Dance, America's Best Dance Contest or sports! ESPN has great for mainstream sports coverage and Fuel TV has amazing coverage of extreme sports like skateboarding, motor cross, surfing, biking, snowboarding, and X-games.

- **Create lists of friends for different activities**. I keep a list of friends with phone numbers next to my desk under different categories like walkers, tennis players, runners, hikers, yoga-lovers. That way when a spur-of-the-moment window of opportunity opens, I just call up a friend without having to think!

- **Switch iPods with a friend.** I highly recommend asking friends to switch! It makes me laugh (listening to some of the songs my friends chose) and gives me inspiration (some great songs that I've never heard before.) I've even cried on runs, when a friend's tune evoked a personal memory. Listening to their playlists is invigorating because it's unpredictable and makes for an interesting workout!

- **Do a burst of exercise** like a quick run up several flights of stairs, or a set of push-ups, as many times a day as needed for stress relief and distraction into present moment awareness. This helps me banish thoughts that dwell on future stress, and gets me back on track taking one task at a time.

- **Get dropped off to run home.** On drives home from errand running or vacations, my boyfriend will pull over 6 miles from our town to let me out. My kids wave at me running along the road. It's fun to reach home an hour later and see everyone there.

- **Bike around town for short errands.** Make it a family affair. Hop on a bike and go to the store, post office, pharmacy. You get the added bonus of reducing emissions and being eco-friendly! It's fun to think about what life would be like without cars!
- **Read Men's Fitness Magazines**. Try adding bits of their harder workouts into yours. I incorporate aspects of strength training from men's plans when mine feel easy or I just want to try something new.

15-minute Night Circuit

Once my kids are in bed, I have a positive routine that keeps me active. I do a 15-minute circuit as I start watching TV. It's restorative and engaging. It increases mobility, flexibility and metabolism. Do each of the 15 activities for 40 seconds and then rest for 20 seconds. (See 'Night Circuit Poses' on page 56 in Appendix.)

1. March with high knees. Hands behind head, knee touches elbows.
2. Cat and dog yoga moves. On hands and knees, swing torso down, looking up, and then round your back up, looking down. Repeat.
3. Downward dog. Palms on floor, arms straight, head looking down, buttocks up towards ceiling, legs straight, feet shoulder width apart, heels stay down. It's like an upside-down 'V.'
4. Wide-straddle squat and hold.
5. Downward dog, again.
6. Wall sit-ups. Place buttocks against wall, legs up on wall, lay on back.
7. Runner's lunges. Lunge forward with left leg, keep left knee beyond ankle, keep right leg straight back, and have both arms pointed straight up to the ceiling.
8. Wall sit-ups, again.
9. Runner's lunges, again, this time with the right leg.
10. Wall sit-ups, again.
11. Arm circles, forward.
12. Wall sit. Place back flat against wall, sit with knees at 90 degree angle, keep feet flat on floor, and hold.
13. Arm circles, backwards.

14. Laying torso twist. Lying down, hold top leg over the bottom leg at waist level. Hold 20 seconds each side.
15. Flat-back foldover. Both arms out straight. Bend at waist with flat back and straight legs, and place hands on the edge of a counter, table or couch arm. Hold for one to two minutes. This is my favorite in the circuit—it really releases weight on my hips. It's so great that I do this one every day, actually, before bedtime.

Commercial-time Exercises

When watching TV at any time of the day, I do some moves during the commercials. Here are my 3 favorite moves.

1. Turn your head all the way to the right and left slowly 10 times.
2. Look at the ceiling for a minute. All day we look down at our computers so your neck muscles are thankful for the change!
3. Hold both arms straight-up to the ceiling for a minute. All day they hang down!

Stay Lighthearted

When I'm in a light-hearted mood, I'm much more able to have a productive life, as well as be less annoyed with anybody or situation.

Here are some tricks I do to get in a good mood:

- **Go to the bathroom**. My dogs run to me whenever I sit on the porcelain thrown and I pet them. They know it's the most opportune time for me to focus my attention on them. (Obviously we're not a close-the-door-to-pee family!) Petting them is cathartic. They are so simple. I imagine going into their heads and feeling their peace.
- **Pretend any chaotic, uncontrollable, annoying situation is part of a film set**. Any difficult situation I face, I simply imagine we're being filmed. I'm an actress, and these pesky people are in the film. They are not really trying to annoy me, in a personal way. They're just there because of the film.
- **Breathe in deeply through my nose** with eyes closed and out through my mouth with eyes open.
- **Fake problem**. This is the quickest and easiest to incorporate into my days. It's a phrase I use

to stop we-have-a-problem thoughts. Since those negative thoughts trigger uncomfortable emotions (and no one likes to feel miserable) I banish those feelings immediately by saying these two words—fake problem. I acknowledge that it's just temporary and can then focus on my health, my lovely family, my great circle of friends, and my good life. If all that's so great, who needs fake problems? They're not real anyway!

- **Perform one stretch**. Stop stressful thoughts with a favorite stretch. Mine is is waterfall yoga pose. Let your head hang down loosey-goosey and try to let go of all neck tension. The head rush from blood changing direction flushes away unwanted thoughts. Okay, maybe that last bit is imaginary, but visualizing it makes the stretch even more impactful.

Enjoy the Week!

I like giving days nicknames, it makes any negative connotations associated with the days much less powerful. Mondays are *Manic Mondays*. Then I have *Tread-water Tuesdays*, *Wonderful Wednesdays* (since it's the one day both my kids have no sports practices or music lessons), *Thankful Thursdays*, and (you guessed it!) *Fantastic Fridays*, which can also be *Fart-astic Fridays* if we ate mom's chili on Thursday. The last two are definitely my favorite weekday names. Then we have *Super-duper Saturdays* and *Sleep-in Sundays*. Ahh! Great, fun names make the week flow by in a wave of positivity and optimism.

Chapter Three:

Diet Tips and Tricks

I love sweets, especially after a good healthy meal. However I know I can't perform solely on sugar. I need protein, calcium, vitamins, minerals, fiber, and healthy carbohydrates along with any sugar! Overall I believe in health. I also believe that calories from any food are usable fuel. So my philosophy is to enjoy my food and balance out my next choices to feel good.

"What is patriotism but the love of the food one ate as a child?"
-Lin Yutang

Health Biography

I was raised with two extremes. My mom was very health conscious, though occasionally she would splurge on sweets. She played tennis weekly. Today, she's still a strong woman. When I was young, she subscribed to wellness newsletters from Stanford and UC Berkeley which documented new trends in medicine and health. I was fed liver and spinach when they were popular sources of iron. Then there came the years of carob when that was suspected to be better than chocolate. Along came the spoonfuls of oat bran when it was announced as something that would add years to our lives.

Candy was restricted at home. I attended the movies with plastic bags of raisins and nuts. But my best friend's house always had cookies and sweets, so I ate much more than my parents knew. (Looks like you can never stop a sugar lover!)

Every chance I got to make homemade cookies, I would. My mom also enjoyed baking, cooking and making dinners. One of her labors of love was making *polechinthas*, traditional Hungarian crepes, with the thinnest batter I'd ever seen. The patience it took to make 40 individual crepes, one by one was admirable. It was in retrospect, later as an adult, that I gained this admiration of her commitment and patience. I recall her standing at the kitchen counter for hours, dipping the crepe maker into the bowl of batter, swirling it around evenly, and waiting for the first signs of bubbles to remove it from the heat. As the stack of crepes grew I could hardly wait to fill them with sweetened cream cheese, top them with her homemade berry compote, and the finishing touch—powdered sugar. After my mom poured some sugar into a small metal strainer, I'd delicately tap and sift the fine fairydust-like sugar through it. It was as pretty as the first snowfall on a mountain.

My dad, on the other hand, enjoyed lots of comfort food like potato chips and sweets. But my mom made sure he ate healthy too. With my Dad, I experienced the delight of cafeteria buffets. He taught me how to use the soup bowl for my ice cream sundae which was much bigger than the little cups by the machine! He was also an avid runner. I remember his lean legs poking out as he headed off for a run. He'd do it all: easy, long, tempo, interval or hill runs.

Another of our beautiful baking traditions occurred on Christmas morning. My dad's mom, Grandma Baker, baked sticky buns every year and we'd wake up to a house full of presents and the aroma of cinnamon sugar. It's really no surprise that my maiden name is Baker!

So with influences from healthy eating to comfort indulgences, I saw how each one made each of my parents happy, and I emerged in between. Needless to say, that both of my parents, with their unique take on food, are alive and kicking!

In junior high and high school, my stay-at-home mom made sure I started the day with a nutritious breakfast. Then at school, I spent my $2 lunch allowance on ding-dongs, mini powdered doughnuts, greasy cheesy rolls, and tater tots. After school I played sports: tennis in the fall, soccer in the winter, swimming in the spring. I'd stay at school until 5 pm practicing sports. Thank goodness I'd always end the day with a well balanced dinner!

Many parents stress out over their kids nutrition. I say if you have healthy choices available at home, take a daily multi-vitamin, stay active and give some sugar-lovin', it's all going to be okay. I eat a healthy diet about 80% of the time, and I feel great! I allow myself sugar because that feels good too. I think if it were restricted from my life it would become a bigger obsession!

All in all, I try to have fun as I'm being responsible. I see myself as the main character in my life's play, amusing myself (and hopefully others) with my activities and sugar-filled moments! I try to lighten up, accept my choices, and then balance out my choices so I feel good. Sometimes balancing out my sugar induced choices involves a healthy streak, so read on...

Eating Styles

I cycle through different eating styles which relate to my eating companion (girlfriends, partner, and kids), my menstrual cycle, and other hormone issues.

I believe balance is the key to everything in life, diet included. People don't generally talk about balancing extremes, just trying to eat balanced meals every day. This, of course, is a good goal. But Native Americans and early settlers, for example, didn't eat perfectly balanced meals day in and day out. They'd eat only meat for months on end without the availability of fruits and vegetables in the winter months.

I applied this logic last 4th of July, when I accepted a request to be in our town's pie eating contest. I like firsts--trying new things is my cup of tea. And when you combine that with sweets, I'm in, no questions asked! Locally-made, world-renowned Olalaberry Pie? Sure, bring it!

I'm competitive, but I really didn't care how I fared. (Well, maybe I did want to beat a few people!) My eating strategy was to eat only the filling, which weighed the most, and it paid off. I ended up scoring 5th place when the pie pans were weighed, out of about 20 eaters! To balance everything, for dinner later that evening, I ate raw broccoli and snap peas with hummus and some plain meat. This way, I got all the categories of the food pyramid.

So, basically, pie contest or not, I tend to cut myself lots of slack. In the spirit of the early settlers, I don't stress out if my daily or weekly intake isn't perfectly in-line with the food pyramid or my physical activity. I never turn down a delicious homemade margarita or dessert at a friend's house. They put their time and energy into making it and part of eating good food is feeling the love that went into making it! Balancing out my choices so that I'm able to enjoy sweets is what keeps my mind engaged.

If I don't eat a balanced meal one day, I'll balance my choices, somehow, in the following days and weeks. Because I have lots of positive habits in place, this helps me meet my goals!

Here are some styles of eating that I find entertaining:

- **Mini good streaks**: My rewarding game is to eat healthy for three days and the fourth day I get to eat whatever I want.
- **Moderation**: Days include checks and balances of the food pyramid in my head. If I eat an apple fritter for breakfast, that's one fruit, one fat and one carb. So, I try to fill in the rest of the pyramid for lunch and dinner (read 'Food Pyramid Guidelines' on page 7).
- **Portion-size**: Focus is on the size of portions at meals. I'll likely eat one "fist-size" portion for breakfast, two portions for lunch and three for dinner.
- **High sugar consumption**: There are days when I eat more carbs and sweets than is needed for basic survival. So, swinging 180 degrees towards a really healthy diet makes up for it. When my mind settles, I go back to eating in moderation.
- **Healthy streak**: Eat the healthiest thing available wherever I am, no sweets. When at my hormonal best this is possible for 14 days. If I'm on a healthy streak, I try to beat my last streak and make it to 15 days. Hasn't happened yet, here's to working towards it!

- **Big dinner style**: Cut breakfast and lunch in half, no snacks, drink water to hold me over and eat a fulfilling dinner and dessert.
- **Eat like a child**: Eat when I'm hungry and eat slowly. Gosh, my kids eat slowly! They talk and talk and talk and if I didn't say, 'Hey, put something on your fork please and let's finish dinner,' they may just hang out at the table for an hour. The upside is: they're my best role models. When I act like them, I feel happy. How simple is that! Take more time at dinner. Eat slower, eat what you crave. I try to put 3 colors of food on their plate each meal. Many nights they'll eat them all, some nights they won't. I'm more consistent with my offerings to them for breakfast and lunch, than I am with myself. So why don't I just copy them all the time? When I do, I feel pretty darn good! This is when I start laughing at myself, at the irony of recognizing a perfect habit, yet not doing it. I chalk it up to my brain needs problems to solve—it's a fake problem!

I remember when my kids were in high chairs. When they were done, they just started smearing, poking and throwing their food. I can laugh now at how irritated I felt at their messiness and how annoyed I felt in having to clean it up. But all in all, I've forgotten the headache because it all turned out fine. Because, they did, after all, grow out of ending their meals in that way!

I think that's how all of life is: messy at times, but turning out fine.

Food Balance

Let's face it, everyone has to watch what they eat. Not many of us can eat whatever we want. It's a known fact that as we age we need less food because our metabolism decreases, which is a major bummer, since I'm constantly learning to cook and bake better!

Overall, I know what I've eaten in a day. I make educated choices to indulge in desserts, skip snacks or lunches some days, cut meal portions in half other days. I guess because I tend to enjoy a lot of variety, I have to keep better track. If you've mastered your diet and rarely get lured off track, this book probably sounds silly. But for those who need the flexibility and variety, having several guideline eating styles, like those listed above, will allow for changing things up while still staying balanced. Anyway, it makes it more fun for me!

Healthy foods boost immune systems, develop bones, increase blood oxygen, and flush out toxins. This is why I love healthy foods. I also love sweet foods because I enjoy the process of creating them—baking, tasting and comparing sweets. Just as a wine enthusiast appreciates varieties of wines and the art of winemaking, I love sweets and baking.

And as it turns out, certain sweets have healthy benefits too. Chocolate, for example, contains polyphenols, which act as antioxidants to help combat oxidative free radicals in our bodies! Chocolate has been shown to have 2x the antioxidant levels of prunes, which have among the highest levels of fruits. And a report from Harvard University found that people who eat sweets, including chocolate, appear to live almost a year longer, on average, than those who do not. Pharmacologists at the Neurosciences Institute in San Diego have also shown that eating chocolate unleashes cannabinoids in the brain, which make us feel happy. Learning these facts helped me feel a lot better about including bits of it in just about anything. Researchers at UC Davis found that 1.5 oz of milk chocolate had similar antioxidant properties as a 5-ounce glass of red wine.

Personally, I feel like it's better to eat sugary sweet things and counterbalance that with health, versus eat a lot of sugar and doing nothing to help your body, or deprive oneself of all sugar and binge eat with guilty conscience. I really do advocate health and also advocate acceptance of sugar in my diet.

Occasionally blending health into my desserts or baking recipes fulfills both of my requirements. Engaging my left brain to modify ingredients and include different portions makes me feel smart like some sort of kitchen scientist! What will happen if I add a package of chopped spinach, use milk instead of water, and add a scoop of protein powder with an extra egg yolk to the box brownie mix? (It actually tastes pretty similar, surprisingly.) How will this pumpkin muffin batter turn out if I smash in half a cup of tofu, add some flax seed and an extra egg? (It turns moist and tasty too!)

Food has a history. When I bake and eat I delve into some subliminal connection to this food history. My foods and my eating habits don't spring out of nowhere, but rather they've developed over time, throughout my life. The memories, the love and the good old fashioned effort of my family and friends emanate through their baking and sharing. It seems unrealistic to strip myself of these beautiful experiences and cut out sugar completely.

There are times where I've reached my caloric necessity or I'm driving 5 hours to see my family, and need something to fiddle with. Sugar-free gum or Ice Breaker Sours help satisfy my sweet tooth. I also get the added bonus of not having to worry about brushing my teeth afterwards!

Get Your Fluids

Did you know your brain is 75% water? So, slight dehydration can cause headaches and worse. Water, water, water is all I can say. Two cups before each meal, one in between each meal and one at bedtime. That's my goal.

I read once that people mistake hunger for thirst. So I tried to be conscious of this; when I thought I was hungry, I drank water, and indeed it actually was true! My displaced feeling of thirst, or what I was interpreting as hunger, would go away with a glass of water. Every time I'm hungry I drink a glass of water or tea and it helps curb my appetite.

I drink V8 regularly for 2 servings of veggies and only 70 calories!

Hot cocoa is the perfect night time drink. It's warm and chocolaty—which is just plain delicious. And it's also kind of healthy! I usually make mine with two tablespoons of cocoa, two tablespoons of sugar, and one cup of skim milk. The total calories equal 150 per cup.

I love tea! Add a little Coffee-mate to any tea and it tastes like a cookie! Also, if you're a tea-lover, try cookie-flavored black tea by Lupicia—it's my new favorite.

I rarely drink juice or soda because I get more enjoyment from consuming baked goods and desserts. Calorie for calorie, I'd just rather sink into a slice of chocolate cake than drink a glass of soda.

And, boy, do I love smoothies! When overripe bananas get to the point when they won't be eaten, I peel and freeze them to use later. Mix one frozen banana, half a cup skim milk, four ice cubes, half a cup of water, one scoop of vanilla whey protein powder and two tablespoons of peanut butter for a delicious drink. This clocks in at about 400 calories. Substitute a cup of blueberries for the peanut butter, and this will bring you in at 300 calories.

Vitamins & Supplements

Here is what I take with my breakfast:

- Multi-vitamin for women
- Calcium, magnesium, zinc, and vitamin D (all in one pill)
- Omega 3 and 6 oils (in two different pills, from flax and fish oils)

As soon as I feel a little sick, I take an Airborne tablet or a powdery vitamin packet with water for a vitamin boost.

For sore muscles, adrenaline pumped days or if I start to feel a little sick, an Epsom salt bath works wonders. Toss two cups of Epsom salt into a warm tub, and soak for 20 minutes while listening to some mellow tunes. Try it out—it's the perfect ending to a hectic day. If curious, search "health benefits of Epsom salt" on-line and read about it's many benefits to the body. Epsom salt is made up of both magnesium and sulfate, which as it turns out, are easier to absorb through our skin vs. a supplement. So, take an Epsom salt bath, and reap the benefits ranging from relieving pain or muscle cramps, to flushing toxins, to improving nerve function and circulatory health, to relieving stress and migraines.

~

For more information on how to integrate a
healthy diet into a busy life, check out
Got Sugar? Recipe Companion.
It's filled with time-saving tips, kitchen guides,
and delicious, quick recipes for
meals, and of course, sweets!

~

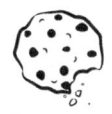

Chapter Four:

Thoughts on Exercise

Exercise burns. Every day, when starting out for the first five to ten minutes, my muscles hurt. It'll be like that until I'm warmed up. I might struggle at first but I keep going. Soon the exercise itself is rewarding enough that there's no need to search for external motivation. And man, does that last set of strength training hurt! But that's not a bad thing because it keeps me in reach of my goals. I know from experience —like after losing all strength and endurance from time off with injuries or pregnancies—that it's always easier to keep up than catch up.

I've trained for years to stay strong and maintain or increase endurance, and completed two marathons in 2009-1010, qualifying for Boston Marathon in 2011. I play co-ed baseball Monday nights two Seasons per year and women's soccer on Sundays. I also competed in the ABC obstacle-course game show "Wipeout" in June of 2010 and won my episode (#303 Anderson Can't Dance.) Bottom line, once I designed and committed to a plan that worked for me, I have felt so motivated to continue since I'm enjoying the benefits of being strong. (I outline the four plans I rotate between in my Workout Companion Book.)

Oddly enough, by stressing my body with exercise, I feel relief! It helps me get away from life when it overwhelms. Exercise calms my mind and I focus better afterwards with less stress. Exercise releases endorphins, which are known to alleviate mild depression. And the physical exertion itself helps me sleep more soundly at night! These reasons are good enough to make me love exercise, but there's more: when I work out, guilt for eating sweets is minimized.

When it gets tough, I still press on. In these cases, even if I don't run or lift weights as hard as I have in the weeks prior, I'll go through the motions at an easier lever and complete the work out in the allotted time. It's my main positive habit that keeps me grounded—so I never stray. I'll never say that I'm too tired for a workout, or that I'll try to make up with extra time tomorrow. On tough days, I'll still exercise, but I'll do it at a lower intensity. I feel good knowing that I didn't bail out. So although I didn't go all out, my confidence is still boosted. Amazing how that works! Just the pride in having exercising boosts my mood and makes me feel good about being strong!

Now that I've built some stamina over time, my legs, feet, tendons and joints have adapted. So I'm able to sustain my workouts more easily before tiring!

> *"The pessimist sees difficulty in every opportunity. The optimist sees the opportunity in every difficulty."*
> -Winston Churchill

Exercise Goals

I strive to maintain mobility, flexibility, and strength in my physical health. Since those three things matter to me, I feel happy working out.

A primary goal is to stay challenged and entertained with my workouts, since I get bored easily. Any diet or exercise regime gets boring. So, I change my schedule four times a year to hold my interest in the game (see 'Seasonal Workout Guide' in *Got Sugar? Workout*

Companion). I also tell myself really important things to keep motivated (see 'Play Games' in *Got Sugar? Workout Companion*).

Though there's definitely something to be said for routine, too much routine makes for a rigid and mundane program. If you aren't flexible, your workouts could get boring and you run the risk of losing interest and motivation. If you're program is too easy, you'll never stay in shape. So it's great to have a foundational structure in which you can easily flex and adapt.

Another goal of mine is to complete an efficient workout: get a good exercise session in the least time. I achieve this by alternating between muscle areas. Previously, I was doing three repetitions of triceps, resting, and then moving on to doing three repetitions of abs and resting again. I was resting for longer in between each set of repetitions, because the muscles hurt from using them three times in a row, and I wasn't able to do as many reps because they were exhausted. By doing what I call a rep-rotation, in which I exercise four different areas in immediate succession, I increase my momentum because I alternate muscle work and can work each area harder with less rest between those reps. (read 'Strength Training Workout Guide' in *Got Sugar? Workout Companion* for more.) I designed this program for myself when the many other methods didn't hold my interest.

> *"I haven't failed, I've just found 10,000 ways that won't work."*
> -Thomas Edison

Visualize!

Each morning I visualize my strength and it makes me smile! If I exercise, I fulfill my goals, and fulfilling goals makes me happy! Visualize yourself doing the work, visualize yourself enjoying the work, and visualize yourself achieving your goals. It creates a positive, can-do mindset, as well as simply motivating you to get started on whatever stands before you.

Say Yes

I try to say yes to everything my kids ask me to play, with a hidden goal to raise my heart rate by playing with them for 10 minutes. If we're on the floor playing kitty, I'll hold a lower pose to work my arms as I make a bridge they can crawl under. If we're on our trampoline we'll see who can do 10 jackknife jumps in a row without falling over. We all try. Falling over and over as we play is all part of the fun, it's hilarious to cheer each other on! Then, when I get back to chores, like fixing dinner or paying bills, that great mood will have carried over. Bursts of action at random times, like playing with my kids, boost my level of playfulness, which keep me young at heart and makes me happy.

"Don't be afraid to go out on a limb. That's where all the fruit is."
-H. Jackson Brown

Why Not!

Another game I play is the 'why not' game. It's invigorating. Just saying 'Sure, why not!' is kind of like saying yes, but it's much more fun. When friends ask me to do things I've never done before like sailing, playing hand ball, helping set up for the school play, mountain biking in an unfamiliar area, I'll give it a try!

Applying this theory socially can really help you challenge your fears. Like doing karaoke—does that activity scare you? Why not just give it a try and see how it goes! The activity and the company are always rewarding (if nothing else, entertaining for your friends and you conquered a fear!)

When a friend asked me to join her on a night run, with a new head light strapped to my forehead, I said, 'Why not!' The experience was great—we saw a few deer, a raccoon and many birds!

When an instructor corrects my position, I don't take it personally, I'm receptive. People might give me advice when they know something I don't. Since it might work, I just say, 'Why not?!' and I'll try it out.

Exercise Tips

Here is a collection of random thoughts pertaining to exercise:

Try running random distances, called *fartlets* in running circles. I do this each week. I'll sprint to the end of my street, for example, or I'll sprint to a car, or I'll race to the mail box across the street and back.

Do twists and turns and lunges to different drawers as I unload the dishwasher. Or try timing yourself to see how fast you can unload it, and then try to beat it next time.

Do a short fast workout if you're short on time. Sprint for 20 seconds and walk 40 seconds, ten times to get your heart beating fast during a workout. Or, run for 15 minutes hard. That's better than walking for 15 minutes, especially if you like to eat sugar like me!

Get a gadget or app. *Fitdeck* Mobile on Blackberries or Fitness Builder on iPhones both offer exercises organized by targeted body areas. It's easy to keep finding new exercises so you don't get bored.

Get a head light so you can run earlier or later, to fit more into your busy day. They usually run about $20, and it's awesome entertainment! I turn my head left, right, slightly up, slightly down to see what I can light up in my path. Pretending there might be a cool animal just around the corner keeps me on my toes, staying ready to sprint away from it if necessary.

Enlist the '40-second on, 20-second off' rule everywhere! As I do laundry, I lift the liquid detergent in my right hand for 40 seconds while loading with my left hand. When volunteering at the grammar school, I park down the street and mini-skip backwards for 40 seconds to the entrance. I pull in my stomach for 40 seconds many times a day, even as I sit in my chair typing this!

Take the stairs. When I'm with my kids, we push the elevator floor button inside and then jump out to run up the stairs. We find it hilarious to see if we can beat the elevator to our floor. If we're stuck waiting for an appointment, we'll go up and down the stairs three more times together and time ourselves. We have fun betting on how much faster we can do it the third time.

When I'm being environmentally aware, I teach my kids that omitting the elevator timing game makes it an eco-friendly choice.

When flying solo, I like to see how well my strength training is working and I trot up the stairs. If I'm really in pain, I'll know that I probably need to work on my quads and do some extra bursting moves!

Exercise in random places. When I walk my dogs to the park, I'll do some yoga moves while they sniff and explore. I'll stretch, move from downward dog to cobra five times, and finish off with some warrior lunges. Initially I was uncomfortable outside at a public park. But after doing it a few times, and having people smile at me, it's made me happy that I challenged my fears and with my physical effort too!

Play with or near kids. Sometimes I grab my kid's skateboard or scooter and just go back and forth in the driveway, or I'll jump rope for 5 minutes while they are outside playing next to me. I wrestle with my son. I get goofy and dance around to some good tunes with them!

Own a big trampoline! I jump four to five times a week with my kids. I try to jump hard for a full minute without stopping, five different times. By jumping in the late afternoon I get an extra mini-burst of feeling strong!

Do micro-exercises while sitting in the car, watching sporting events, or waiting at the doctor's office. Performing these mini-moves twice a week challenges my mind to remember how many sets I did before getting interrupted. It not only gets you moving, but it also makes the time fly by!

Micro-exercises

I aim to do each move for 40 seconds, 3 times. I pulse them to the beat of the music!

- **Butt cheek clenches**: I make up variations like double-time for 8 beats, on the beat for 8, double-time for 8, on beat for 8, double-time for 8, and that's 40 seconds up!
- **Leg clenches:** Tighten tops of upper leg to the beat of the song.
- **Hand clenches:** With hands on the wheel at 2 and 10 o'clock, tighten fists into a clench.

- **Elbow squeeze**: With hands on the wheel at 2 and 10 o'clock, squeeze elbows in towards each other. Pulse or hold in as long as you can.
- **Toe scrunches:** These help build arch strength. You can do them while in cruise control in the car, or while sitting in a chair waiting.
- **Toe tapping**: This builds shin strength. You can also do these while in cruise control in the car, or while sitting in a chair waiting.
- **Heel raises:** These work your calves. Do these while in cruise control in the car, or while sitting in a chair waiting.
- **Tighten inner thighs**: Put a book, bottle of water or whatever item in between legs and hold.
- **Kegel muscle tightening:** Do this to the beat of the music!
- **Neck resisting**: Push on each side of head above ear, and resist. Push back against headrest, push on forehead with one hand. These are four different positions that are great to alternate and hold.
- **Waist wiggle**: Tighten stomach and move waist side-to-side to the beat.
- **Pull stomach in:** Flatten your back against the seat and pull your stomach muscles in.

- **One arm punch**: This is great to do to a rock song. Do it hard, so you feel it! It'll make another driver smile at you!

Structure is good, but occasionally toss out the workout plan! Do something new or different, faster or slower. It's great for mental health as well. For example, during the summer when I swim more, I'll drop the arm portion of the weight sets in the same week. Think of ways to change the exercise, while keeping in mind what muscles you want to work to keep a balance of arms, legs and core.

I try to keep doing more active things every day, not less. This way my body has a reason to use the sugary things I consume!

Injury Prevention Ritual

One of the most important things about getting healthy, is staying healthy. To do this, you need to stay injury-free. Injuries hurt, they zap time, and with an injury I can't move around as much. This means, I have less opportunity to use up the energy I've consumed.

So, each morning, to gear up for a day of movement, I perform a mini warm up. It's like a little injury prevention ritual that I do before I get out of bed. Do each of the following for 20 seconds:

1. Roll ankles.
2. Bicycle legs.
3. Straighten legs, flex and hold them up to the ceiling.
4. Slowly open and close legs for easy inner thigh and hip movement.
5. Hip stretch, crossing left leg over the right, grab left knee with right hand and hold. Then switch.
6. Sit up on bed side and roll neck. Look up, down, left, right.

Then when I stand up I've got some juices lubricating my joints and I'm ready for more movement.

Also good posture means better alignment and less chance of injury from favoring a side. So when you sit in a chair at work, try not to lean one way or the other. Sit straight and engage your back and stomach muscles to hold your torso erect.

And finally, to prevent injury, I <u>don't do the same thing two days in a row</u>. Different exercises stimulate different muscles, and there'll be less chance of overusing them and causing injury!

I do what works for me, modifying moves or positions to keep going. Variety is great! If my hip hurts, I'll skip parts of the workout that use my hip and focus on things that don't use it: I'll do more core and arm work until it's healed. I keep exercising but I modify the movements. Sometimes to prevent injury, I need to go at a slower speed.

And don't forget, drink water! Water lubricates connective tissue, which helps prevent injury!

Always remember to focus on where you're going, instead of where you've been!

~

For more information on workout tips
that inspire, check out
Got Sugar?
Workout Companion.
It's complete with body areas,
exercise guides, strength training
suggestions, and annual
workout plans.

~

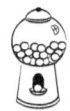

APPENDIX

Night Circuit Poses

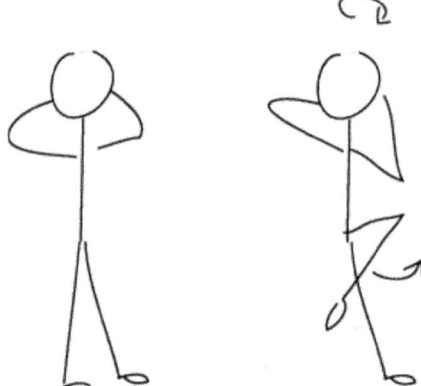

1. March with High Knees

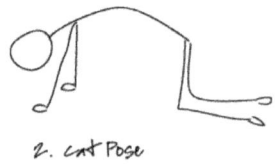

2. Cat Pose

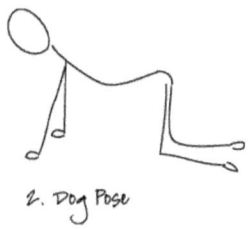

2. Dog Pose

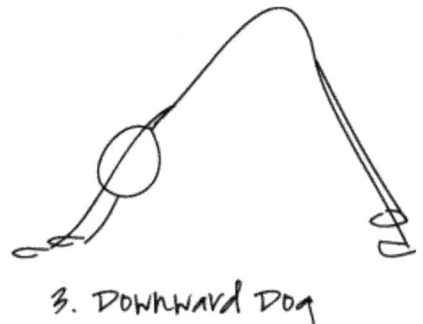

3. Downward Dog

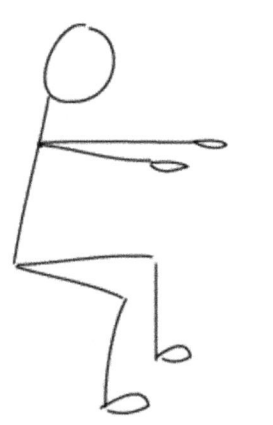

4. Wide-straddle Squat

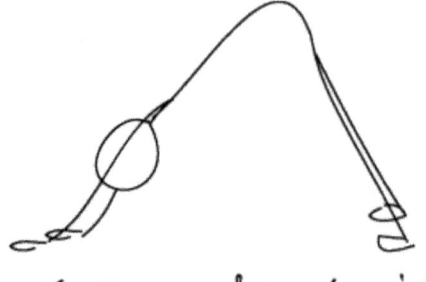

5. Downward Dog (again)

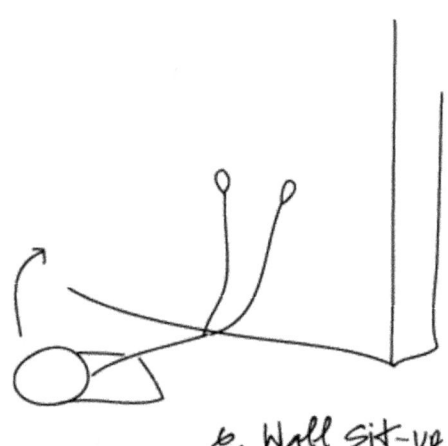

6. Wall Sit-up

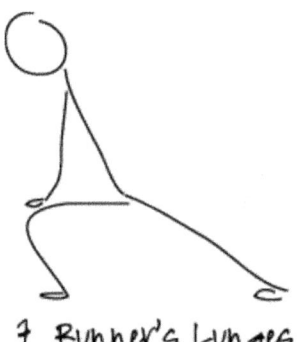

7. Runner's Lunges

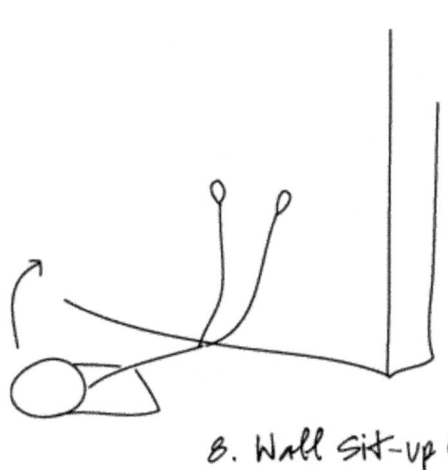

8. Wall Sit-up (again)

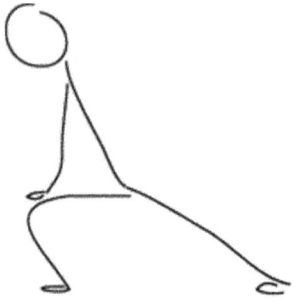

9. Runner's Lunges

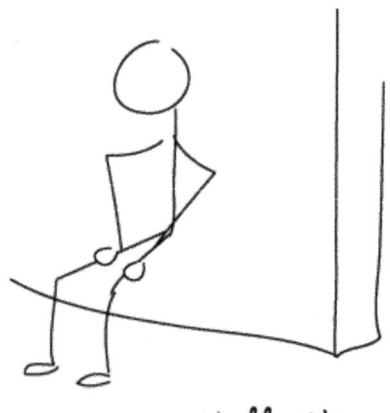

10. Wall Sit

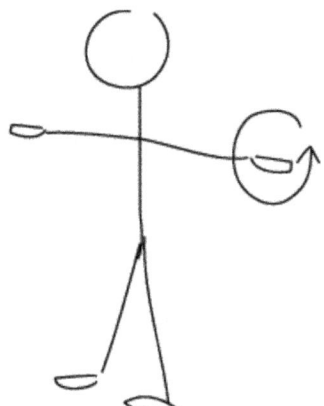

11. Arm circles (forward)

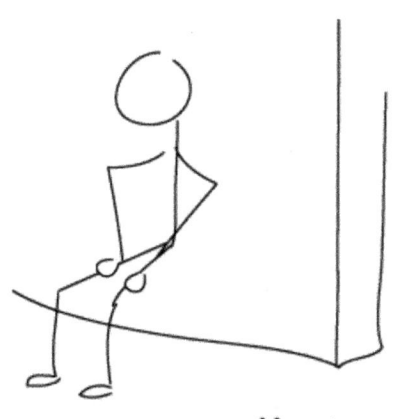

12. Wall sit (again)

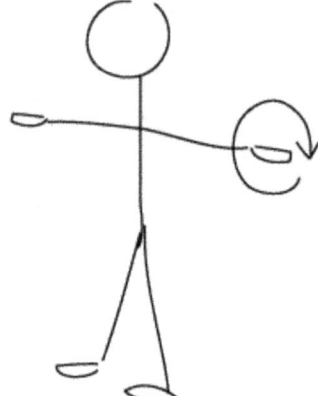

13. Arm circles (backward)

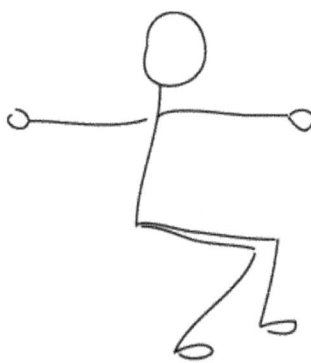

14. Lying Torso Twist
(aerial view)

15. Flat-back Foldover

~

Share your thoughts or feedback! Tell me the things you love, any health and fitness tips or family recipes and I'll post them in my blog!

~

Connect with Debbie Online:

Facebook: Functionably Happy

Blog and Website: www.functionablyhappy.com

email: debbie@functionablyhappy.com